NAVIGATING KIDNEY FAILURE

A Comprehensive Guide to Managing Your Health and Resources

TABLE OF CONTENTS

INTRODUCTION 4
   OVERVIEW OF KIDNEY FAILURE 5
   WHAT ARE THE SYMPTOMS OF KIDNEY FAILURE?. 7
   WHAT HEALTH PROBLEMS CAN PEOPLE WITH KIDNEY DISEASE DEVELOP? 9
   HOW CAN THE PATIENT LIVE WELL IF HE HAS KIDNEY FAILURE? 11

FIRST STEPS AFTER DIAGNOSIS 13
   TREATING THE CAUSE OF YOUR KIDNEY INJURY 15
   TREATING COMPLICATIONS UNTIL YOUR KIDNEYS RECOVER 15

LIFESTYLE AND HOME REMEDIES 17

WHAT IS NEPHROLOGY? 18
   WHAT DOES NEPHROLOGY STUDY? 19
   WHAT SHOULD BE BRINGING TO THE CONSULTATION OF A NEPHROLOGIST? 21
   IMPORTANCE OF CONSULTING A NEPHROLOGIST 22
   WHEN TO SEE A NEPHROLOGIST 25
   INITIAL TESTS AND ASSESSMENTS 26
   UNDERSTANDING YOUR TREATMENT OPTIONS ... 27

NAVIGATING YOUR HEALTH CARE 29
   INSURANCE COVERAGE 29
   HOW TO CHECK WHAT YOUR INSURANCE COVERS 31
   TIPS FOR DEALING WITH INSURANCE COMPANIES 32

DIALYSIS: WHAT YOU NEED TO KNOW 38
   TYPES OF DIALYSIS 38
      WHAT IS HEMODIALYSIS? 38
      PERITONEAL DIALYSIS 40
      HOME DIALYSIS 41
CHOOSING A DIALYSIS CENTER 43
   PREPARING FOR YOUR FIRST DIALYSIS SESSION
   49
KIDNEY TRANSPLANTATION 51
   WHEN IS A KIDNEY TRANSPLANT INDICATED? 52
      HOW TO GET ON THE TRANSPLANT LIST 54
LIVING DONORS VS. DECEASED DONORS 56
   LIVING DONORS 56
   DECEASED DONORS 58
   FACTORS TO CONSIDER 59
   SUPPORT AND RESOURCES 61
   LOCAL AND ONLINE SUPPORT GROUPS 62
   EDUCATIONAL RESOURCES AND PATIENT
   ADVOCACY 64
COPING STRATEGIES AND MAINTAINING MENTAL HEALTH 65
GLOSSARY OF TERMS 69
DEFINITION FOR NEPHROSCLEROSIS 72
FOCAL SEGMENTAL GLOMERULOSCLEROSIS 74
   TYPES OF FSGS 74
POLYCYSTIC KIDNEY DISEASE 76
APPENDIX 78

LIST OF NEPHROLOGISTS AND DIALYSIS CENTERS
....78
LINKS TO SOCIAL SECURITY AND INSURANCE
RESOURCES 80
ABOUT THE AUTHOR **82**
BACKGROUND AND EXPERIENCE 82

INTRODUCTION

Welcome to "Navigating Kidney Failure: A Comprehensive Guide to Managing Your Health and Resources."

This guide is designed to support you from the moment you receive a diagnosis of kidney failure, providing you with essential information, practical advice, and resources to manage your condition effectively.

Receiving a diagnosis of kidney failure can be overwhelming and fraught with uncertainty. The journey ahead may seem daunting, with new medical terms, treatments, and decisions to make about your healthcare. However, with the right knowledge and resources, you can take control of your health and navigate this challenging time with confidence.

This eBook aims to empower you by demystifying kidney failure. We'll explain what kidney failure means, explore the causes and symptoms, and provide a clear pathway for the steps you should take following your diagnosis. You will learn how to work effectively with healthcare professionals, understand your treatment options, and discover how to access the necessary healthcare services.

Additionally, we recognize the importance of support during this time. As such, we'll guide you to resources for emotional and social support and help you connect with communities and organizations that can assist you in your journey.

Our goal is to ensure that you do not feel alone in this. With this comprehensive guide, we hope to equip you with the tools you need to face kidney failure with resilience and informed confidence. Let's take this first step together.

OVERVIEW OF KIDNEY FAILURE

Kidney failure is transient or permanent kidney damage that results in loss of normal kidney function. There are two different types of kidney failure: acute and chronic. Acute kidney failure begins suddenly and is potentially reversible. Chronic kidney failure progresses slowly over at least three months and can lead to permanent kidney failure. The causes, symptoms, treatments, and consequences of acute and chronic kidney failure are different.

Kidney failure, also known as renal failure, occurs when the kidneys lose their ability to perform their essential functions effectively. The kidneys are vital organs that filter waste products, excess water, and other impurities from the blood. These waste products are then excreted from the body in your urine. In addition to filtering waste, the kidneys regulate salt, potassium, and acid content, produce hormones that manage blood pressure, and control the production of red blood cells.

There are two primary forms of kidney failure: acute and chronic:

- ❖ Acute Kidney Failure occurs suddenly, often within a few days or weeks. It can be reversible with immediate and appropriate treatment. Causes include severe dehydration, a rapid loss of blood, and certain acute infections.

- ❖ Chronic Kidney Disease (CKD) progresses more slowly and is usually caused by long-term conditions that put a strain on the kidneys. Common causes include high blood pressure, diabetes, and inherited conditions. Unlike acute kidney failure, CKD is often not reversible and can lead to permanent kidney damage over time.

When the kidneys fail, harmful levels of fluid and waste can accumulate in the body, leading to potentially life-threatening complications. Early stages of kidney failure may be managed with medication and lifestyle changes, but more advanced stages may require treatments such as dialysis or a kidney transplant.

WHAT ARE THE SYMPTOMS OF KIDNEY FAILURE?

Symptoms of kidney failure can start so slowly that the person does not notice them immediately.

Healthy kidneys prevent the accumulation of toxins and excess fluids in the body and balance salts and minerals in the blood, such as calcium, phosphorus, sodium, and potassium. The kidneys also make hormones that help control blood pressure, make red blood cells, and keep bones strong.

Kidney failure means that the kidneys no longer function well enough to perform these functions, and as a result, other health problems occur. As kidney function decreases, the person may:

- swelling, usually in feed, feet, or ankles
- have headaches
- feel itchy
- feeling tired during the day and having trouble sleeping at night
- feeling sick to your stomach, losing your sense of taste, feeling in appetence, or

LOSING WEIGHT

- produce little or no urine
- feeling muscle cramps, weakness, or numbness
- feeling pain, stiffness, or fluid in the joints
- feeling confused, having concentration problems, or memory problems

Following the treatment plan can help prevent or treat most of these symptoms. The treatment plan may include regular dialysis treatments or a kidney transplant, a special eating plan, physical activity, and medications

WHAT HEALTH PROBLEMS CAN PEOPLE WITH KIDNEY DISEASE DEVELOP?

Kidney disease can cause other health problems. The healthcare team will work with the patient to help them avoid or control:

High blood pressure can be both a cause and a result of kidney disease. It damages damaged kidneys, which are less efficient at controlling blood pressure. With kidney failure, the kidneys cannot get rid of excess water. Drinking too much water can cause swelling, raise blood pressure, and make your heart work harder.

Medications to lower blood pressure, limiting sodium and fluids in the diet, staying physically active, controlling stress, and quitting smoking can help control blood pressure.

HEART DISEASE. Kidney disease and heart disease share two of the exact leading causes: diabetes and high blood pressure. People with kidney disease are at high risk for heart disease, and people with heart disease are at high risk for kidney disease.

Measures taken to control kidney disease, blood pressure, cholesterol, and blood glucose (if the person has diabetes) will also help prevent heart attacks or strokes.

ANEMIA. When the kidneys are damaged, they stop producing enough erythropoietin (EPO), a hormone that helps make red blood cells. Red blood cells carry oxygen from the lungs to other parts of the body. When you have anemia, some organs, such as the brain and heart, may get less oxygen than they need and stop working as well as they should. A person with anemia may feel weak and without energy.

The healthcare provider may prescribe iron supplements. In some cases, you may be prescribed medications that help the body make more red blood cells.

MINERAL AND BONE TRASTONE. Healthy kidneys balance calcium and phosphorus levels in the blood and make hormones that help keep bones strong. As kidney function decreases, the kidneys:

They produce less of the hormone that helps the body absorb calcium. Like the domino effect, low calcium concentrations in the blood cause parathyroid hormone to be released. This hormone moves calcium from the bones to the blood. Excess parathyroid hormone can also cause itching.

They stop removing so much phosphorus. Excess phosphorus in the blood also draws calcium from the bones.

Without treatment, bones can wear out and weaken, and the person may feel pain in the bones or joints. Changes in the eating plan, medications, supplements, and dialysis can help.

HOW CAN THE PATIENT LIVE WELL IF HE HAS KIDNEY FAILURE?

Living well if you have kidney failure is challenging. The patient will feel better if:

- Complies with its treatment program
- Check your medications with the healthcare provider at each visit and take them as prescribed

- Works with a dietitian to develop a feeding plan that includes foods that you enjoy eating and are also beneficial to health
- Stay active: go for a walk or do some other physical activity that you enjoy
- Keeps in touch with friends and family

Dialysis or transplant treatment will help the patient feel better and live longer. The health care team will work with the patient to create a treatment plan that addresses any health problems they have. The treatment will include the measures you can take to maintain your quality of life and level of activity.

The feeding plan plays an important role. When a person has kidney failure, what they eat and drink can help them maintain a healthy balance of salts, minerals, and fluids in the body.

Detecting kidney failure early can be challenging, as the symptoms might only appear once the condition has progressed significantly. Regular check-ups are crucial, especially if you are at higher risk due to conditions like diabetes or high blood pressure.

Understanding kidney failure and recognizing its potential causes and symptoms is the first step in managing this condition. With careful monitoring and treatment, many people with kidney failure continue to lead full and active lives. This guide will further explain how to navigate the medical system, manage symptoms, and access the resources you need to support your health journey.

FIRST STEPS AFTER DIAGNOSIS

Receiving a diagnosis of kidney failure can be overwhelming. However, taking the right steps immediately can help you manage the condition effectively. Here are the crucial first steps to undertake following a diagnosis of kidney failure:

You might have the following tests to diagnose acute kidney injury:

BLOOD TESTS. A sample of your blood may show fast-rising levels of urea and creatinine. This helps show how your kidneys are working.

Urine output measures. Measuring how much urine you pass in 24 hours may help find the cause of your kidney failure.

URINE TESTS. A sample of your urine may show something that suggests a condition that might explain kidney failure. This is called urinalysis.

IMAGING TESTS. Imaging tests such as ultrasound and CT scans can show your kidneys.

REMOVING A SAMPLE OF KIDNEY TISSUE FOR TESTING. Your healthcare professional may suggest removing a small sample of your kidney tissue for lab testing. This is called a biopsy. A needle put through your skin and into your kidney removes the sample.

Treatment for acute kidney injury most often means a hospital stay. Most people with acute kidney injury are already in the hospital. How long you'll stay in the hospital depends on the reason for your acute kidney injury and how quickly your kidneys recover.

TREATING THE CAUSE OF YOUR KIDNEY INJURY

Treatment for acute kidney injury involves finding the illness or injury that damaged your kidneys. Your treatment depends on the cause. It might involve stopping a medicine that's damaging your kidneys.

TREATING COMPLICATIONS UNTIL YOUR KIDNEYS RECOVER

Your healthcare team also works to prevent complications and give your kidneys time to heal. Treatments that help prevent complications include:

- **TREATMENTS TO BALANCE FLUIDS IN YOUR BLOOD.**

If a lack of fluids in your blood is the cause of your acute kidney injury, you may need fluids through a vein called intravenous (IV) fluids.

If acute kidney injury causes you to have too much fluid, this may lead to swelling in your arms and legs. Then, you may need medicines called diuretics, which help your body get rid of extra fluids.

✣ MEDICINES TO CONTROL BLOOD POTASSIUM.

Your kidneys need to filter potassium from your blood better. Potassium regulates blood pressure and other body functions.

You might need medicines called potassium binders to keep potassium from building up. These include sodium zirconium cyclosilicate (Lokelma) or patiromer (Veltassa). Too much potassium in the blood can cause irregular heartbeats, called arrhythmias, and muscle weakness.

✣ MEDICINES TO RESTORE BLOOD CALCIUM LEVELS.

If the levels of calcium in your blood drop too low, you might need to get calcium through a vein called an infusion.

Treatment to remove poisons from your blood. If wastes build up in your blood, you may need hemodialysis for a time. Also called dialysis, it helps remove poisons and excess fluids from your body while your kidneys heal.

✛ DIALYSIS ALSO MAY HELP REMOVE EXCESS POTASSIUM FROM YOUR BODY.

During dialysis, a machine pumps blood out of your body through an artificial kidney, called a dialyzer, which filters out waste. The blood is then returned to your body.

LIFESTYLE AND HOME REMEDIES

During your recovery from acute kidney injury, a special diet can help support your kidneys and limit the work they must do. Your healthcare team may send you to a dietitian. A dietitian can look at what you eat and suggest ways to make your diet easier on your kidneys.

YOUR DIETITIAN MAY SUGGEST THAT YOU:

Choose foods lower in potassium. These include apples, peaches, carrots, green beans, white bread, and white rice. Eat them instead of foods higher in potassium, such as potatoes, bananas, tomatoes, oranges, beans, and nuts.

Don't eat foods with added salt. This includes many packaged foods, such as frozen dinners, canned soups, and fast foods. Other foods with added salt include salty snack foods, canned vegetables, and processed meats and cheeses.

Limit phosphorus. Phosphorus is a mineral found in foods such as dark-colored sodas, milk, oatmeal, and bran cereals. Too much phosphorus in your blood can weaken your bones and cause your skin to itch.

As your kidneys improve, you may no longer need a special diet, but healthy eating is still important.

WHAT IS NEPHROLOGY?

Nephrology is a medical specialty dedicated to the diagnosis and treatment of kidney disease. This specialty is oriented to prevention and diagnosis, which allows us to carry out early detection and care for patients affected by kidney pathologies, who tend to suffer a rapid deterioration in their quality of life.

WHAT DOES NEPHROLOGY STUDY?

Nephrology focuses solely on the study of kidney pathologies, so it should not be confused with urology, which treats disorders that affect all organs of the urinary system. Primary and secondary glomerulopathies: These diseases affect the structure and function of the glomerulus, although later, other kidney structures can be implicated. We are talking about primary Glomerulonephritis, when the clinical manifestations are restricted to the kidney, and secondary Glomerulonephritis, when the involvement is within a systemic disease such as lupus, rheumatoid arthritis, etc.

- ❖ **CHRONIC KIDNEY DISEASE**: Chronic kidney disease is considered the final destination of a series of pathologies that affect the kidney chronically and irreversibly. Once the diagnostic and therapeutic measures of primary kidney disease have been exhausted, it can evolve into chronicity, so early action is of vital importance.

- **CARDIONEPHROLOGY:** a high percentage of patients with chronic heart failure have kidney disease. This unit works in the study and in the joint approach of both pathologies.

- **ONCONEPHROLOGY:** On the one hand, kidney patients with dialysis treatment have an increased risk of cancer. On the other hand, cancer therapies can affect the kidneys. This subspecialty allows doctors to have a global vision to treat patients who present these pathologies combined.

- **GERIATRIC NEPHROLOGY** cares for older patients over 70 who, due to the passage of time and a higher incidence of systemic diseases, tend to manifest kidney diseases more frequently.

- **DIAGNOSTIC AND INTERVENTIONAL NEPHROLOGY:** Ultrasound monitoring, puncture and action on fistulas for hemodialysis, placement of a venous catheter for hemodialysis, and ultrasound-directed renal biopsy.

❖ **RENAL SURGERY:** focuses on the surgical treatment of kidney conditions in conjunction with the Urology team.

WHAT SHOULD BE BRINGING TO THE CONSULTATION OF A NEPHROLOGIST?

We recommend that you prepare for the visit, which will be of great help to the doctor. It is advisable to come with a list of symptoms, medications being taken, and relevant history for the case. If you have previous diagnoses or test results, it is also important to remember them.

A few days before the consultation, you will receive a questionnaire to indicate your background, regular medication, and other specific questions that allow us to anticipate some aspects of the consultation. This will help us streamline and offer you much more personalized assistance. For this, we recommend downloading our free application from the

Quirónsalud Patient Portal, which will facilitate communication with your healthcare team.

IMPORTANCE OF CONSULTING A NEPHROLOGIST

EXPERT GUIDANCE: A nephrologist is a physician who specializes in kidney care and is critical in diagnosing and managing kidney diseases. Consulting a nephrologist ensures that you receive expert guidance tailored to your specific condition.

COMPREHENSIVE MANAGEMENT: Nephrologists can coordinate your overall treatment, including the management of symptoms, complications, and the underlying causes of kidney failure. They work in collaboration with other healthcare professionals to provide holistic care.

Consulting a nephrologist, a specialist in kidney care, is crucial for several reasons:

⁜ EARLY DETECTION OF KIDNEY PROBLEMS

Nephrologists are trained to identify kidney issues early, even when symptoms are not apparent. Early detection can prevent further deterioration and improve the long-term outlook.

⁜ SPECIALIZED KNOWLEDGE AND TREATMENT

Nephrologists have extensive knowledge of kidney diseases and are equipped to provide specialized care that general practitioners may need to become more familiar with. This includes managing conditions such as chronic kidney disease (CKD), acute kidney injury (AKI), and Glomerulonephritis.

⁜ MANAGEMENT OF CHRONIC CONDITIONS

For chronic conditions like CKD, nephrologists provide ongoing care and management. This includes monitoring kidney function, prescribing appropriate medications, and recommending lifestyle changes to slow disease progression.

✚ DIALYSIS AND TRANSPLANTATION

Nephrologists play a critical role in managing patients who need dialysis or are candidates for kidney transplantation. They ensure patients receive the right type of dialysis and manage all aspects of pre-and post-transplant care.

✚ PREVENTION OF COMPLICATIONS

Kidney disease can lead to complications such as high blood pressure, anemia, and bone disease. A nephrologist can help prevent and manage these complications, improving the patient's overall quality of life.

✚ PERSONALIZED CARE

Nephrologists provide personalized treatment plans based on the patient's specific condition, lifestyle, and overall health. This individualized approach ensures more effective management and better outcomes.

✤ EDUCATION AND SUPPORT

Nephrologists educate patients about their condition, treatment options, and lifestyle modifications. They provide support and resources to help patients manage their condition and maintain a good quality of life.

✤ COORDINATION WITH OTHER HEALTHCARE PROVIDERS

Nephrologists work closely with other healthcare providers to ensure comprehensive care. This collaboration is essential for managing patients with complex medical conditions that affect the kidneys.

WHEN TO SEE A NEPHROLOGIST

Abnormal Kidney Function Tests: Elevated creatinine or blood urea nitrogen (BUN) levels.

- Protein or Blood in Urine: Indicating potential kidney damage.

- Hypertension: High blood pressure that is difficult to control.
- Diabetes: Especially if there is evidence of kidney involvement.
- Family History: Of kidney disease or conditions affecting the kidneys.
- Recurring Kidney Stones: Frequent episodes of kidney stones may require specialized management.

Consulting a nephrologist ensures that you receive expert care for any kidney-related issues, which can significantly improve your health outcomes.

INITIAL TESTS AND ASSESSMENTS

BLOOD AND URINE TESTS: These tests help assess kidney function and are vital for determining the severity of kidney failure. Common tests include serum creatinine, blood urea nitrogen (BUN), and glomerular filtration rate (GFR), which indicate how well your kidneys are filtering waste.

IMAGING TESTS: Ultrasounds, CT scans, or MRIs can be used to check the size and structure of the kidneys, looking for abnormalities that might have contributed to kidney failure.

KIDNEY BIOPSY: In some cases, a biopsy may be necessary to determine the exact cause of kidney failure by examining a small tissue sample from the kidney under a microscope.

UNDERSTANDING YOUR TREATMENT OPTIONS

LIFESTYLE MODIFICATIONS: Changes in diet, exercise, and possibly restrictions on fluid intake can help manage the symptoms and progression of kidney failure. A dietitian may be involved in creating a personalized eating plan.

MEDICATIONS: Depending on the cause and stage of kidney failure, medications might be prescribed to help control symptoms, manage complications, and slow progression. These can include blood pressure medications, diuretics, or erythropoietin to prevent anemia.

DIALYSIS: If kidney function is significantly impaired, dialysis might be required to help remove waste products and excess fluid from the blood. There are two main types: hemodialysis and peritoneal dialysis.

KIDNEY TRANSPLANT: This is a surgical option where a healthy kidney from a donor replaces the failing kidney. Transplantation is often considered the most effective treatment for restoring kidney function and improving quality of life.

SUPPORT SERVICES: Psychological counseling, support groups, and patient education programs can be integral to managing the emotional and practical challenges of kidney failure.

Taking these initial steps after being diagnosed with kidney failure is crucial for setting a positive course for your treatment and management of the disease. It empowers you with the knowledge and resources needed to tackle kidney failure proactively and optimally.

NAVIGATING YOUR HEALTH CARE

Managing kidney failure involves:

- Navigating various aspects of healthcare.
- Particularly understanding.
- Utilizing your insurance coverage effectively.

Here's how you can manage your healthcare needs through your insurance:

INSURANCE COVERAGE
UNDERSTANDING YOUR INSURANCE PLAN

First and foremost, it's essential to understand the details of your health insurance policy. Review your plan to determine what types of kidney-related treatments and medications are covered. Check for any exclusions, limitations, and prior authorization requirements. This knowledge helps you avoid unexpected costs and ensures that you receive the necessary care without unnecessary delays.

It's crucial to have a clear understanding of what your health insurance covers, especially when it comes to treating chronic conditions like kidney failure. Coverage can vary widely depending on whether you have private insurance, Medicare, or another type of health plan.

Key Aspects to Review in Your Insurance Plan:

DIALYSIS AND TREATMENT: Check if your plan covers both hemodialysis and peritoneal dialysis and what kind of coverage it offers for kidney transplants.

MEDICATIONS: Ensure that your insurance covers the medications commonly prescribed for kidney failure, including those to manage complications and comorbidities.

SPECIALIST VISITS: Since regular visits to a nephrologist are essential, confirm that these are covered and understand the referral process if required by your insurer.

ADDITIONAL THERAPIES: Some plans may cover additional therapies like nutritional counseling, which can be crucial for managing kidney failure.

HOW TO CHECK WHAT YOUR INSURANCE COVERS

✦ CONTACT YOUR INSURANCE PROVIDER

The most direct way to understand your coverage is to contact your insurance provider. Most insurers provide a customer service number that you can call for detailed information about what is covered and what your responsibilities are in terms of co-pays and deductibles.

✦ REVIEW YOUR POLICY DOCUMENTS

Your insurance policy documents provide detailed information about coverage limits, the types of services covered, and the procedures for filing claims and disputes. Regularly reviewing these documents can help you stay informed about your coverage.

✦ USE ONLINE RESOURCES

Many insurance companies offer online portals where you can access your insurance information, check coverage details, and sometimes even chat online with customer service for clarifications.

TIPS FOR DEALING WITH INSURANCE COMPANIES

BE PROACTIVE

It's important to be proactive and not wait until a crisis occurs. Understanding your coverage in advance can save you significant time and stress later.

KEEP GOOD RECORDS

Keep detailed records of all your healthcare visits, treatments, and correspondence with your insurance company. This documentation is essential if you need to dispute a claim or clarify your coverage.

ASK QUESTIONS

If you're you need clarification on any aspect of your coverage, ask questions. It's better to get clarifications directly from your insurer to avoid surprises, especially about what treatments and medications are approved and the extent of coverage for each.

SEEK ASSISTANCE

If navigating your insurance coverage becomes overwhelming, consider seeking help from a social worker, patient navigator, or financial counselor within the healthcare system. These professionals can provide guidance and support in dealing with insurance issues.

STAY INFORMED ABOUT CHANGES

Insurance policies can change, and so do laws that affect healthcare coverage. Stay informed about any changes in your insurance policy or health laws that might affect your coverage.

Navigating your healthcare effectively through your insurance is crucial in managing kidney failure. It ensures that you can access the necessary treatments without undue financial stress, allowing you to focus more on your health and less on bureaucratic complexities.

IN-NETWORK PROVIDERS AND FACILITIES

To maximize your insurance benefits and minimize out-of-pocket costs, it's important to seek care from in-network providers and facilities. These are healthcare professionals and institutions that have agreements with your insurance company to provide services at negotiated rates. Find out which nephrologists, dialysis centers, and hospitals are in-network, and build your treatment plan around these providers.

COVERAGE FOR MEDICATIONS

Kidney failure often requires a regimen of medications to manage symptoms and complications. Verify which medications are covered by your insurance plan and whether they are included in the formulary list. Additionally, check if your plan covers generic versions of your medications, as these can be more cost-effective. If a prescribed medication is not covered, speak with your healthcare provider about alternatives that are covered by your insurance.

DIALYSIS AND TRANSPLANTATION COSTS

Understanding the associated costs and insurance coverage is crucial for patients requiring dialysis or a kidney transplant. Dialysis can be a significant financial burden, so knowing the extent of coverage, co-pays, and any additional costs can help you plan better. For kidney transplants, insurance typically covers the surgery, hospitalization, and post-operative care, but it's essential to confirm these details and understand any specific requirements or limitations in your policy.

PREVENTIVE CARE AND REGULAR MONITORING

Preventive care and regular monitoring are vital in managing kidney failure. Many insurance plans cover preventive services, such as blood tests, urine tests, and routine check-ups, which can help detect and address complications early. Take advantage of these covered services to stay on top of your health and prevent further deterioration of kidney function.

COORDINATION WITH HEALTHCARE PROVIDERS

Effective communication and coordination with your healthcare providers can streamline the management of your condition and optimize the use of your insurance benefits. Ensure that your nephrologist and other specialists are aware of your insurance details so they can make informed decisions about your care and refer you to in-network providers when necessary.

FINANCIAL ASSISTANCE PROGRAMS

In cases where insurance coverage is insufficient, explore financial assistance programs offered by non-profits, government agencies, and pharmaceutical companies. These programs can help cover costs for medications, treatments, and other healthcare needs related to kidney failure. Additionally, some hospitals and dialysis centers offer financial counseling services to help you navigate these options and reduce the financial strain.

APPEALS AND ADVOCACY

If you encounter denied claims or coverage issues, don't hesitate to appeal the decision. Insurance companies have processes for appealing denied claims, and providing additional documentation or a letter from your healthcare provider can often overturn these decisions. Advocacy organizations for kidney disease patients can also provide support and guidance in navigating the appeals process and ensuring you receive the coverage you need.

Managing kidney failure effectively requires a thorough understanding of insurance coverage and proactive planning to fully utilize your benefits. By staying informed, coordinating with your healthcare providers, and seeking financial assistance when needed, you can better manage the financial aspects of your treatment and focus on maintaining your health and well-being.

DIALYSIS: WHAT YOU NEED TO KNOW

Dialysis is a lifesaving treatment for those with kidney failure. It helps the kidneys function by removing waste, salt, and extra water to prevent them from building up in the body. It also helps maintain a safe level of certain chemicals in the blood and controls blood pressure. Understanding the types of dialysis, choosing the right center, and preparing for your sessions are essential steps.

TYPES OF DIALYSIS

DIALYSIS AND HEMODIALYSIS

Dialysis treats end-stage renal failure. This procedure removes waste from the blood when the kidneys can no longer do their job.

WHAT IS HEMODIALYSIS?

The main function of your kidneys is to remove toxins and extra fluid from the blood. If waste products accumulate in the body, it can be dangerous and even cause death.

Hemodialysis (and other types of dialysis) fulfills the function of the kidneys when they stop working well.

Hemodialysis can:

- Eliminate extra salt, water, and waste products so they don't build up in your body.
- Maintain safe levels of minerals and vitamins in your body
- Help control blood pressure
- Help make red blood cells

During hemodialysis, blood passes through a tube to an artificial kidney or filter.

The filter, called a dialyzer, is divided into 2 parts separated by a thin wall.

As the blood passes through one part of the filter, a special liquid in the other part removes the residue from the blood.

The blood then returns to the body through a tube.

The doctor will create an access where the tube connects. Usually, access will be in a blood vessel in the arm.

HEMODIALYSIS

- ❖ **HOW IT WORKS**: Hemodialysis involves circulating your blood through a machine, which cleans it before it is returned to your body. A minor surgery is usually needed to create vascular access, which is an entry point in your body to access your bloodstream.

- ❖ **FREQUENCY**: This type of dialysis is typically done three times a week, each session lasting about four hours, although more frequent, shorter sessions are becoming common.

- ❖ **SETTING**: It can be performed in a hospital, a dialysis center, or at home with proper training and equipment.

PERITONEAL DIALYSIS

- ❖ **HOW IT WORKS**: Peritoneal dialysis uses the lining of your abdomen, called the peritoneum, and a unique solution called dialysate to absorb waste and fluid from your blood. The dialysate is put into your abdomen through a catheter, absorbs waste, and is then drained away.

❖ **FREQUENCY**: This can be done daily or multiple times a day, depending on the method used (Continuous Ambulatory Peritoneal Dialysis or Automated Peritoneal Dialysis).

❖ **SETTING**: Peritoneal dialysis is generally done at home, making it a more flexible option for many patients.

HOME DIALYSIS

You may be able to have hemodialysis at home. You don't have to buy a machine. Medicare or your health insurance will pay most or all of the costs of your treatment at home or in a facility.

- If dialyzed at home, you can use one of these two schedules:
- Shorter treatments (2 to 3 hours), at least 5 to 7 days per week
- Longer treatments at night, 3 to 6 nights per week while sleeping

- You can also do a combination of daily and night treatments.

Since you get treatment more often and it happens more slowly, hemodialysis at home has some benefits:

Helps keep your blood pressure lower. Many people no longer need blood pressure medications.

- It does a better job of waste disposal.
- It is more benign for your heart.
- You may have fewer symptoms from dialysis, such as nausea, headaches, cramps, itching, and tiredness.
- You can more easily accommodate treatments within your schedule.

You can get the treatment yourself, or you can have someone to help you. An expert dialysis nurse can train you and your caregivers on how to do dialysis at home. Training can take anywhere from a few weeks to a few months. Both you and your caregivers should learn to:

- Manage the team
- Place the needle at the access site

- Control the machine and your blood pressure during treatment
- Keep records
- Clean the machine
- Order supplies, which you can receive at home

Dialysis at home is only for some. You have a lot to learn and must be responsible for your care. Some people feel more comfortable having a provider to handle their treatment. Also, not all centers offer dialysis at home.

Dialysis at home can be a good option if you want more independence and are able to learn how to do the treatment yourself. Talk to your provider. Together, they can decide what type of hemodialysis is right for you.

CHOOSING A DIALYSIS CENTER

Choosing a dialysis center is a significant decision for individuals with kidney failure, as it directly impacts their quality of care and overall well-being. Here are some key considerations and steps to help you make an informed choice:

⁕ LOCATION AND ACCESSIBILITY

The location of the dialysis center is a crucial factor. Ideally, the center should be conveniently located near your home or workplace to minimize travel time and stress. Consider the availability of transportation options, such as public transit, shuttle services provided by the center, or parking facilities if you drive.

⁕ QUALITY OF CARE

Research the quality of care provided by potential dialysis centers. Look for centers with high ratings from national or state health organizations, such as the Centers for Medicare & Medicaid Services (CMS) in the United States. These ratings can give you an idea of the center's performance in areas like patient outcomes, infection control, and overall care quality.

⁕ STAFF EXPERTISE AND SUPPORT

The expertise and support of the staff at the dialysis center are vital. Ensure that the center is staffed with experienced nephrologists, nurses, dietitians, and social workers who can provide comprehensive care.

Additionally, observe the staff's demeanor and willingness to answer questions during your visit. A supportive and knowledgeable team can greatly enhance your dialysis experience.

✤ FACILITY CLEANLINESS AND SAFETY

Visit the dialysis centers you are considering to assess their cleanliness and safety protocols. A clean, well-maintained facility is essential for preventing infections and ensuring a comfortable treatment environment. Ask about the center's infection control measures and how they handle emergencies or complications during dialysis sessions.

✤ DIALYSIS SCHEDULE AND FLEXIBILITY

Consider the dialysis center's schedule and its flexibility to accommodate your lifestyle. Dialysis treatments are typically required multiple times a week, so it's important to find a center that offers appointment times that fit your daily routine. Some centers provide evening or weekend sessions, which can be beneficial for those with work or family commitments.

✦ TREATMENT OPTIONS

Different dialysis centers may offer varying treatment options, including in-center hemodialysis, home hemodialysis, and peritoneal dialysis. Evaluate which treatment method is best suited for your medical condition and lifestyle. If you prefer home dialysis, ensure the center provides adequate training and support for at-home treatments.

✦ PATIENT EDUCATION AND SUPPORT PROGRAMS

A good dialysis center should provide patient education and support programs. These programs can help you better understand your condition, manage your treatment, and improve your overall health. Look for centers that offer classes, support groups, and individual counseling to address the emotional and psychological aspects of living with kidney disease.

⊹ FINANCIAL CONSIDERATIONS

Understand the costs associated with treatment at each dialysis center and what your insurance will cover. Some centers may offer financial counseling services to help you navigate insurance benefits and explore options for financial assistance if needed. Make sure the center you choose is in-network with your insurance plan to minimize out-of-pocket expenses.

⊹ PATIENT REVIEWS AND TESTIMONIALS

Seek out reviews and testimonials from current or former patients of the dialysis centers you are considering. Their experiences can provide valuable insights into the quality of care, the environment, and the staff's professionalism. Online reviews, patient forums, and word-of-mouth recommendations can all be useful sources of information.

⁜ COMMUNICATION AND COORDINATION WITH HEALTHCARE PROVIDERS

Choose a dialysis center that communicates effectively and coordinates with your primary care physician and other healthcare providers. This ensures a seamless exchange of information and continuity of care, which is crucial for managing your overall health and any comorbid conditions.

⁜ EMERGENCY PREPAREDNESS

Inquire about the dialysis center's emergency preparedness plans. Understanding how the center handles power outages, natural disasters, or other emergencies can give you peace of mind, knowing that your care will continue uninterrupted in any situation.

By carefully considering these factors and thoroughly researching your options, you can choose a dialysis center that meets your medical needs, fits your lifestyle, and provides the highest quality of care.

QUESTIONS TO ASK:

- What is the patient-to-nurse ratio?

- How flexible are the scheduling options?
- What kind of support services are available (dietary advice, social work, etc.)?

PREPARING FOR YOUR FIRST DIALYSIS SESSION

PHYSICAL PREPARATION:

- ❖ **Medical Check-Up**: Before starting dialysis, a complete medical check-up is often required to assess your overall health and any specific needs during dialysis.

- ❖ **UNDERSTAND THE PROCEDURE**: Familiarize yourself with the dialysis process. Knowing what to expect can help alleviate anxiety.

WHAT TO BRING:

- ❖ **COMFORT ITEMS**: Such as a blanket, pillow, and something to occupy your time like books, headphones, music, or a tablet.

- ❖ **MEDICAL INFORMATION**: Bring a list of your current medications and any recent test results.

- ❖ **SNACKS**: Check with the center if you can bring snacks or a meal, especially since sessions can last several hours.

MENTAL PREPARATION:

- ❖ **Mental Health Support**: It's normal to feel overwhelmed or anxious. Consider speaking to a counselor or joining a support group to share your feelings and receive support from others who understand your experience.

By understanding the types of dialysis, choosing the right center, and preparing adequately for your sessions, you can manage your kidney failure more effectively, leading to a better quality of life despite the challenges.

KIDNEY TRANSPLANTATION

A kidney transplant is a surgery in which a healthy kidney is transplanted into a person with kidney failure. In order to do it, a kidney donated by a healthy individual is needed, and it can come from a living donor, related or not to the patient, or from a deceased person. The option of a transplant from a living donor is valid since only one kidney is necessary to replace the function of both, but it must be compatible.

Kidney transplantation is a critical treatment option for those with end-stage renal disease (ESRD) or severe kidney failure. It involves surgically placing a healthy kidney from a donor into a patient whose kidneys no longer function properly. This section covers the transplant process, how to get on the transplant list and the differences between living and deceased donors.

WHEN IS A KIDNEY TRANSPLANT INDICATED?

Not all people are transplant candidates. About a fifth of dialysis patients have access to transplantation for medical or other reasons.

Each candidate's study is personal. For example, age is not a priori an exclusion criterion since transplants are performed on younger children and people of very advanced ages.

The improvement in survival and quality of life of the patient requires a previous study that identifies:

- The patient's state of health.
- That the transplant is technically feasible.
- Demographic and risk factors.
- Comorbidities that determine the suitability of the patient.

Immunity and psychosocial situations must be minimized to minimize pre- and post-operative complications to be included in the transplant waiting list (LE).

Some counter-indications regarding transplant access prevent people from being included on the waiting list. Once the condition of limited access has been overcome, however, the person may be included.

THE TRANSPLANT PROCESS EXPLAINED

EVALUATION AND APPROVAL: Before you can receive a transplant, you must undergo a thorough evaluation to determine if you are a good candidate for surgery. This includes physical exams, blood tests, and assessments of your mental and emotional health to ensure you can handle the surgery and the post-transplant regimen.

FINDING A DONOR: Once approved, the search for a suitable donor begins. This can be a living donor (typically a family member, friend, or an altruistic donor) or a deceased donor (someone who has chosen to donate their organs upon death).

SURGERY: When a donor kidney is found, the transplant surgery is scheduled quickly. The procedure generally lasts several hours, during which the donor's kidney is placed in the lower abdomen and connected to blood vessels and the bladder.

RECOVERY: After surgery, you will spend several days to weeks in the hospital. The new kidney may start working right away or may take some time to begin functioning. Doctors will monitor for any signs of rejection or infection.

POST-TRANSPLANT CARE: Following discharge, frequent follow-ups and medication adjustments are necessary to prevent organ rejection and manage side effects. Lifelong medications to suppress the immune system and to avoid rejection are required.

HOW TO GET ON THE TRANSPLANT LIST

REFERRAL BY A NEPHROLOGIST: Your nephrologist must refer you to a transplant center for evaluation.

TRANSPLANT CENTER EVALUATION: The center conducts a series of tests to determine if you are a suitable candidate for transplantation.

REGISTRATION: If approved, your details are added to a national transplant waiting list, such as the one managed by the United Network for Organ Sharing (UNOS) in the United States.

WAITING PERIOD: The waiting time for a donor's kidney can vary significantly, often several years, depending on your blood type, health status, and availability of matching donors.

LIVING DONORS VS. DECEASED DONORS

Choosing between a living donor and a deceased donor for a kidney transplant is a crucial decision that impacts the outcome and overall success of the transplant. Here's a detailed comparison of the two options:

LIVING DONORS

❖ **ADVANTAGES:**

Better Outcomes: Kidneys from living donors tend to function better and last longer compared to those from deceased donors. This is because the kidney is removed and transplanted quickly, minimizing the time it spends outside the body.

Shorter Waiting Time: Patients receiving a kidney from a living donor can avoid the long wait on the transplant list. This is particularly beneficial as the waiting time for a deceased donor kidney can be several years.

Scheduled Surgery: The transplant surgery can be scheduled at a convenient time for both the donor and the recipient, allowing for better planning and preparation.

Pre-Transplant Compatibility Testing: There is the opportunity to conduct thorough pre-transplant testing to ensure the best possible match between the donor and recipient, reducing the risk of rejection.

Immediate Function: Kidneys from living donors often start functioning immediately after the transplant, whereas kidneys from deceased donors may take some time to "wake up" and start working.

- ❖ **DISADVANTAGES**:

Risk to the Donor: The donor must undergo major surgery, which carries risks such as infection, bleeding, and potential complications. There is also a psychological impact on the donor.

Availability: Finding a suitable living donor can be challenging. Not everyone has a family member or friend who is willing and able to donate a kidney.

Emotional and Ethical Considerations: The process can be emotionally complex for both the donor and recipient and ethical considerations regarding the donor's health and well-being may exist.

DECEASED DONORS

❖ ADVANTAGES:

No Risk to Living Individuals: The kidney comes from a recently deceased person, so there are no risks associated with living donation.

Greater Pool of Donors: Deceased donation increases the availability of kidneys, offering hope to those who do not have a living donor option.

Equitable Distribution: National transplant organizations manage the allocation of deceased donor kidneys, ensuring a fair and equitable distribution based on medical needs and compatibility.

❖ DISADVANTAGES:

Longer Waiting Time: The waiting time for a deceased donor kidney can be lengthy, often several years, which can be challenging for patients on dialysis.

Potential for Delayed Function: Kidneys from deceased donors may not start working immediately after the transplant, sometimes requiring dialysis until the kidney "wakes up."

Lower Overall Success Rates: While still effective, kidneys from deceased donors generally have slightly lower success rates and shorter longevity compared to those from living donors.

Urgency of Surgery: Once a deceased donor kidney becomes available, the transplant must be performed quickly, which can be logistically challenging and stressful.

FACTORS TO CONSIDER

Health and Compatibility: The health of both the donor and recipient and their compatibility are critical factors. Living donors undergo extensive health evaluations to ensure they can safely donate a kidney.

Ethical and Emotional Considerations: The decision to accept a kidney from a living donor involves significant ethical and emotional considerations. It's essential to ensure that the donor is fully informed, willing, and not coerced into donating.

Medical Urgency: The severity of the recipient's condition and the urgency of the transplant can influence the choice between a living and deceased donor.

Support and Resources: The availability of support systems and resources for both the donor and recipient plays a crucial role. Post-transplant care, emotional support, and financial resources are important considerations.

Personal Preferences: The preferences and values of the recipient and their family, including their willingness to wait for a deceased donor or accept the risks and benefits of a living donation, are fundamental in making this decision.

Both living and deceased donor kidney transplants have their unique advantages and disadvantages. The choice between the two depends on various factors, including the recipient's health, the availability of a living donor, and the urgency of the transplant. Consulting with healthcare professionals, including nephrologists and transplant coordinators, can help recipients and their families make an informed decision that best suits their needs and circumstances.

Kidney transplantation can dramatically improve the quality of life for individuals with severe kidney failure. Understanding the process, preparing for the possible waiting period, and considering all donor options are essential steps in this life-changing journey.

SUPPORT AND RESOURCES

Navigating life with kidney failure is not just about managing physical health but also about addressing emotional and social needs. Support and resources are crucial for providing patients and their families with the knowledge, assistance, and community needed to handle the challenges of kidney disease. Here's a guide to finding support and accessing valuable resources:

LOCAL AND ONLINE SUPPORT GROUPS

LOCAL SUPPORT GROUPS

- ❖ **BENEFITS**: Local support groups offer a chance to meet others facing similar challenges, exchange practical advice, and share emotional support in a face-to-face setting. These groups can also provide connections to local resources and healthcare professionals.
- ❖ **FINDING THEM**: Hospitals, community centers, and organizations like the American Association of Kidney Patients and the National Kidney Foundation often host or direct you to local support groups.

ONLINE SUPPORT GROUPS

- ❖ **BENEFITS**: They offer flexibility and accessibility, particularly for those who may be geographically isolated or have mobility issues. Online forums and social media groups can provide 24/7 access to support.

- ❖ **Finding Them**: Websites like ☐ PatientsLikeMe, ☐ HealthUnlocked, or specific Facebook groups dedicated to kidney health can be excellent platforms.

EDUCATIONAL RESOURCES AND PATIENT ADVOCACY

EDUCATIONAL RESOURCES

PURPOSE: Understanding kidney failure and its management can empower patients, reduce anxiety, and help them make informed health decisions.

RESOURCES: Reputable sources include the

- American Association of Kidney Patients,
- National Kidney Foundation
- American Kidney Fund, and
- NIHClearinghouse&Health Information Center, which offer pamphlets, videos, and detailed guides about treatments and lifestyle management.

PATIENT ADVOCACY

ROLE OF ADVOCATES: Patient advocates help navigate healthcare systems, access medical services, and understand patient rights.

ACCESSING ADVOCACY SERVICES: Many hospitals provide patient advocates, or you can contact organizations like the Patient Advocate

Foundation for support in dealing with insurance issues, medical bills, and treatment access.

COPING STRATEGIES AND MAINTAINING MENTAL HEALTH

Mental health IS health. It includes your emotional, psychological, and social well-being and impacts how you think, feel, act, and relate to others. The tools below can play an important role in maintaining positive mental health and supporting treatment and recovery of mental health if you have a mental health condition.

✤ EAT WELL

Eating well helps you function well. It can also increase your energy and mood, feed your brain, and reduce the risk of developing certain diseases.

✤ HELP OTHERS

Helping others can help you feel less depressed and calmer, increase your happiness, feel connected and needy, and add a purpose to your life.

✢ SLEEP ENOUGH

Sleeping enough and of good quality can help decrease the risk of depression and anxiety, decrease the risks of certain diseases, improve your memory, and, in general, improve your feeling of well-being.

✢ CONNECT WITH OTHERS

We often turn to our friends and loved ones for support, especially in times of stress. This can increase happiness, lower blood pressure, help us feel supported and valued, and help us live longer.

✢ BE PHYSICALLY ACTIVE

Exercise can help prevent heart disease and high blood pressure, reduce the risk of certain diseases, improve sleep and increase energy, decrease stress levels, anger, tension, anxiety, and depression, and improve the feeling of well-being.

✢ FOCUS ON THE POSITIVE.

Having negative thoughts can affect your mood, your actions, and even your physical health. Focus on the positive as much as possible.

✢ FIND JOY IN YOUR LIFE.

Finding joy and happiness can help decrease pain, stress, and anxiety, as well as develop emotional strength.

USING COPING SKILLS DURING DIFFICULT TIMES

We all experience moments of additional stress, but having coping skills can help you feel less stressed and depressed and manage the stressful times.

GET PROFESSIONAL HELP IF YOU NEED IT.

Never be afraid to ask for help. If your mental health problems prevent you from working or feeling well, professional help can make a big difference.

COPING STRATEGIES

- **Routine**: Establishing a daily routine can provide a sense of normalcy and control.
- **Physical Activity**: Engaging in proper physical activities can improve both physical health and emotional well-being.

- ❖ **Hobbies and Interests**: Maintaining hobbies and interests can help divert focus from illness and enhance quality of life.

MENTAL HEALTH MAINTENANCE

- ❖ **Professional Support**: Therapists or counselors specialized in chronic illness can help address feelings of depression, anxiety, and stress.
- ❖ **Mindfulness and Relaxation Techniques**: Practices like meditation, yoga, and deep-breathing exercises can reduce stress and improve overall mental health.

FAMILY AND FRIENDS

- ❖ **Involving Loved Ones**: Educating friends and family about kidney failure and how they can support can strengthen personal relationships and provide additional emotional support.

These resources and strategies are essential for building a supportive network and maintaining mental and emotional health while managing kidney failure. With the right support, patients can more effectively navigate the complexities of their condition and lead fuller, more satisfying lives.

GLOSSARY OF TERMS

Navigating kidney failure involves understanding various medical and insurance-related terms. This glossary provides definitions of common terms that patients may encounter during their treatment and management of kidney disease.

MEDICAL TERMS

- **Albuminuria**: The presence of albumin, a type of protein, in the urine, is an early sign of kidney damage.
- **Creatinine** is a waste product produced by muscle metabolism; high levels in the blood can indicate impaired kidney function.
- **Dialysis**: A medical procedure that removes waste products and excess fluid from the blood when the kidneys can no longer do so effectively on their own.
- **Erythropoietin**: A hormone produced by the kidneys that stimulates the bone marrow to produce red blood cells.

- **Glomerular Filtration Rate (GFR)**: A test that measures the level of kidney function and determines the stage of kidney disease.
- **Hemodialysis**: A type of dialysis that uses a machine and a filter to clean the blood; typically performed in a clinic or hospital.
- **Nephrologist**: A physician who specializes in the treatment of kidney diseases.
- **Peritoneal Dialysis**: A type of dialysis that uses the lining of your abdominal cavity to filter your blood.
- **Renal**: Pertaining to the kidneys.
- **Uremia**: A condition resulting from the buildup of waste products in the blood due to impaired kidney function, characterized by nausea, fatigue, and a metallic taste in the mouth.

INSURANCE TERMS

- **Co-pay**: A fixed amount paid by a patient for a covered healthcare service, typically paid when receiving the service.
- **Deductible**: The amount a patient needs to pay out-of-pocket before the insurance company starts to pay its share of the costs.

- **Exclusion**: Specific conditions or circumstances that are not covered by an insurance policy.
- **Formulary**: A list of prescription drugs covered by a prescription drug plan or another insurance plan offering prescription drug benefits.
- **Network**: The facilities, providers, and suppliers your health insurer has contracted with to provide health care services.
- **Out-of-Pocket Maximum**: The most you have to pay for covered services in a plan year. After you spend this amount on deductibles, co-payments, and co-insurance, your health plan pays 100% of the costs of covered benefits.
- **Premium**: The amount that must be paid for your health insurance or plan. You and your employer usually pay it monthly, quarterly, or yearly.
- **Prior Authorization:** A requirement that your physician obtain approval from your health insurance plan to prescribe a specific medication or service.

> **Provider**: Any healthcare professional, hospital, or health service organization that provides healthcare treatment.

Understanding these terms can help patients more effectively manage their health care and navigate the complexities of insurance policies. This knowledge empowers patients to make informed decisions about their treatment options and financial responsibilities.

DEFINITION FOR NEPHROSCLEROSIS

Nephrosclerosis is a medical condition characterized by the hardening (sclerosis) of the small blood vessels in the kidneys. This condition can lead to reduced blood flow to the kidneys and subsequently impair their function. There are two main types of nephrosclerosis:

❖ **BENIGN NEPHROSCLEROSIS**

This type is associated with long-standing hypertension (high blood pressure) and ageing.

- It typically progresses slowly and may not cause significant kidney damage for many years.
- It is characterized by hyaline arteriolosclerosis, where the walls of the small arteries and arterioles thicken and become hyalinized (glassy)

❖ MALIGNANT NEPHROSCLEROSIS:

This more severe form is associated with malignant hypertension, which is an extreme and rapid increase in blood pressure.

- It progresses quickly and can lead to significant kidney damage and failure.
- It is characterized by hyperplasic arteriolosclerosis, where the walls of the small arteries and arterioles undergo a proliferative thickening, often leading to an "onion-skin" appearance.

Symptoms of nephrosclerosis can vary depending on the severity and type. Still, they may include signs of chronic kidney disease such as hypertension, proteinuria (protein in the urine), and reduced kidney function. Treatment often involves managing blood pressure and other underlying conditions to slow the progression of kidney damage.

FOCAL SEGMENTAL GLOMERULOSCLEROSIS

Focal segmental glomerulosclerosis (FSGS) is a disease in which scar tissue develops on the glomeruli, the small parts of the kidneys that filter waste from the blood. Various conditions can cause FSGS.

FSGS is a severe condition that can lead to kidney failure, which can only be treated with dialysis or a kidney transplant. Treatment options for FSGS depend on the type you have.

TYPES OF FSGS

- **PRIMARY FSGS.**

Many people diagnosed with FSGS have no known cause for their condition. This is called primary (idiopathic) FSGS.

❖ SECONDARY FSGS.

Several factors, such as infection, drug toxicity, diseases including diabetes or sickle cell disease, obesity, and even other kidney diseases, can cause secondary FSGS. Controlling or treating the underlying cause often slows ongoing kidney damage and might lead to improved kidney function over time.

Genetic FSGS is a rare form of FSGS caused by genetic changes. It is also called familial FSGS. It's suspected when several family members show signs of FSGS. Familial FSGS can also occur when neither parent has the disease, but each carries a copy of an altered gene that can be passed on to the next generation.

In some cases, the underlying cause of FSGS cannot be determined despite evaluating clinical symptoms and extensive testing.

SYMPTOMS

Symptoms of focal segmental glomerulosclerosis (FSGS) might include:

- Swelling is called oedema in the legs and ankles, around the eyes and other body parts.

- Weight gain from fluid buildup.
- Foamy urine from protein buildup is called proteinuria.

POLYCYSTIC KIDNEY DISEASE

Polycystic kidney disease (PKD) is an inherited disorder in which clusters of cysts develop primarily within the kidneys, causing them to enlarge and lose function over time. Cysts are noncancerous round sacs containing fluid. They vary in size and can grow very large. Having many or large cysts can damage the kidneys.

Polycystic kidney disease can also cause cysts to develop in your liver and elsewhere in your body. The disease can cause serious complications, including high blood pressure and kidney failure.

PKD varies significantly in its severity, and some complications are preventable. Lifestyle changes and treatments might help reduce damage to your kidneys from complications.

SYMPTOMS

Polycystic kidney disease symptoms can include:

- High blood pressure
- Back or side pain
- Blood in your urine
- A feeling of fullness in your abdomen
- Increased size of your abdomen due to enlarged kidneys
- Headaches
- Kidney stones
- Kidney failure
- Urinary tract or kidney infection

APPENDIX

This section provides useful links and contact information to help patients access nephrologists, dialysis centers, transplant hospitals, and resources related to Social Security and insurance. While this guide does not list individual contacts due to variability by region and changes over time, it directs you to where to find these resources effectively.

LIST OF NEPHROLOGISTS AND DIALYSIS CENTERS

Finding a Nephrologist:

- **American Society of Nephrology (ASN)**: Offers a directory of nephrologists across the United States. ASN Website

- **American Association of Kidney Patients (AAKP)**: Are dedicated to improving the quality the quality of life for kidney patients through education, advocacy, patient engagement, and the fostering of patient communities. AAKP Website

- **National Kidney Foundation (NKF)**: Provides a search tool to find kidney doctors based on location. NKF Physician Finder

LOCATING DIALYSIS CENTERS:

- **Dialysis Finder by DaVita**: Enables patients to find dialysis centers near them in the U.S. DaVita Dialysis Center Finder

- **Fresenius Kidney Care**: Another resource for finding dialysis centers across the country. Fresenius Clinic Finder

CONTACT INFORMATION FOR TRANSPLANT HOSPITALS

U.S. Transplant Centers:

- **United Network for Organ Sharing (UNOS)**: Provides a comprehensive list of all transplant centers in the U.S. You can search by state, organ, or center name. UNOS Organ Transplant Regional Resources

INTERNATIONAL TRANSPLANT CENTERS:

- **Transplant Living**: Offers information about international transplant centers. This site can be a starting point for non-U.S. residents. Transplant Living Website

LINKS TO SOCIAL SECURITY AND INSURANCE RESOURCES

SOCIAL SECURITY RESOURCES:

- **Social Security Administration (SSA)**: The official site for Social Security benefits, including disability claims. SSA Official Website

- **Disability Benefits Help**: Provides information on how to apply for Social Security Disability benefits. Disability Benefits Help Site

INSURANCE INFORMATION:

- **HealthCare.gov**: Useful for understanding and choosing health insurance plans, especially during open enrollment periods. HealthCare.gov

- **Medicare**: Official U.S. government site for Medicare. Includes coverage and plan information. Medicare Official Site

These resources are essential for accessing specialized care and understanding the benefits and services available to patients with kidney failure. They can help in making informed decisions about treatment options and managing the costs associated with care.

ABOUT THE AUTHOR

DAVID RODRIGUEZ

David Rodriguez is a distinguished member of the American Association of Kidney Patients (AAKP) and former Patient Relationship Specialist at the University Transplant Institute in San Antonio, TX. With a profound commitment to advancing kidney health and patient rights, David has devoted his career to enhancing the lives of those affected by kidney disease. David is also a kidney and liver transplant recipient

BACKGROUND AND EXPERIENCE

Education: In 2007, David attended St. Edwards University in Austin, TX

Professional Experience: Over the years, David has worked in the healthcare system at the <u>University Transplant Institute – University Hospital</u>, particularly focusing on nephrology and transplant services. His roles have included dialysis clinical visitation centers, patient advocacy, and strategic planning in patient referrals, all within high-profile hospital settings in organ transplantation and patient advocacy organizations.

Advocacy and Leadership: At the American Association of Kidney Patients, David has been instrumental in policy advocacy, striving to ensure that kidney patients receive comprehensive care and support. He has been a vocal advocate for patient rights, actively taking part in legislative efforts to improve healthcare access and treatment options for kidney disease patients.

Contributions to Patient Education: David has authored many articles and patient advocacy focused on kidney and liver health, treatment options, and patient empowerment. His work aims to demystify complex medical information, making it accessible and understandable for patients and their families.

Community Involvement: Beyond his professional endeavors, David is deeply involved in community outreach programs to educate the public about kidney health, prevention of kidney disease, and the importance of organ donation.

RECOGNITION AND AWARDS

David's dedication and commitment to the kidney patient community have been recognized with several awards, including, AAKP's, U.S. Presidential Volunteer Service Award, and Texas Organ Sharing Alliance, Joan Wish Award for Central Region and TePxas Kidney Foundation, Volunteer of the Year Award. His ongoing efforts to improve patient care standards and promote kidney health continue to make a significant impact in the field.

David Rodriguez's extensive experience, combined with his passion for patient advocacy, makes him a respected voice in the kidney health community. His leadership and educational efforts have been crucial in advancing the interests and well-being of kidney patients across the nation.

www.ingramcontent.com/pod-product-compliance
Lightning Source LLC
Chambersburg PA
CBHW071949210526
45479CB00003B/873